Men

How To Fight The Symptoms Of Menopause, No Medication, Natural Solutions, Diet, Secrets And Simple Tips That You Can Apply NOW

Dr. Melissa Keane

Table of Contents

Introduction

I want to thank you and congratulate you for purchasing the book, *"Menopause - How To Fight The Symptoms Of Menopause, No Medication, Natural Solutions, Diet, Secrets And Simple Tips That You Can Apply NOW"*.

There are literally thousands of women reaching menopause every day and, despite the fact that we are currently flooded with lots of information about menopause, many women still have endless questions concerning menopause. Indeed, this can be a very confusing and uncomfortable point in time, plagued with harsh symptoms.

You want to understand better what is going on with your body just before and during menopause so that you can feel better. You may have even been told that the only answer to your troubling symptoms is prescription drugs. As a woman who has personally experienced this, I want to tell you my experience with menopause, what menopause entails and show you great options available for treating your symptoms.

Having trustworthy facts at your disposal will help end any fear, confusion or worry you may be experiencing now. I believe after reading this book, you'll feel empowered and ready to conquer this seemingly scary monster, menopause.

Thanks again for purchasing this book. I hope you enjoy it!

Dr. Melissa Keane

BONUS CHECKLIST!

I know that you are a busy and successful woman. Sometimes, we don't have enough time to check everything and as a result we get stressed. For this reason, I recently created a one-page sheet with my top tips on how to stay in control with menopause. All my best tips packed in one page. To Get Instant Access open a browser and navigate to the short linked page **http://bit.ly/2u1djoo**. Once you download, print it and use it as a quick reference along with this book.

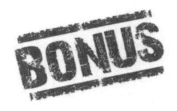

Enjoy,

Dr. Melissa Keane

Menopause Basics

Before we go any further, let us look closely at menopause so that you can have a better understanding of what you are going through.

All women (except transgender women) experience menopause at some point as they age. Menopause generally describes the changes that you go through either just before or after your menses stop, marking the end of your childbearing days.

We (women) are born with a limited number of eggs (oocytes) stored in our ovaries. The ovaries also produce hormones estrogen and progesterone, which regulate menstruation and ovulation. Each year, your ovaries release eggs, until there are no more eggs left- you literally 'run out' of eggs. An end in egg production makes your estrogen and progesterone levels start falling; in some women, it's gradual while others sudden.

It's this fall in estrogen that is linked to many menopausal symptoms. In short, when your ovaries run out of eggs, menopause begins. Therefore, menopause can be redefined as a time in your life as a woman when your ovaries literally "run out" of eggs and not when your periods stop. You see, menopause does not start until 12 months after you stop having periods, when menopause associated symptoms begin. Menopause normally starts at around 45 to 50 years but some of us experience menopause earlier than that, a condition called premature menopause.

How Does Natural Menopause Occur?

Menopause that happens naturally, without any surgeries or procedures goes through three stages:

Perimenopausal; normally starts a couple of years before menopause, when the ovaries start producing less estrogen. It lasts up until menopause at which point the ovaries stop releasing the eggs. Estrogen levels drop faster during the last 1 to 2 years of premenopausal. You start experiencing symptoms at this stage.

Menopause; if it's been a year since you got your menses, then you have reached menopause. At this point, your ovaries have stopped producing eggs and estrogen is very little.

Post-menopausal; this happens years past menopause. In this stage, most of the menopause related symptoms such as hot flashes disappear for most of us. However, as women age, our health risk related to estrogen loss rises.

As earlier mentioned, premature menopause can happen in some people; therefore, let us look at what causes this.

What Causes Premature Menopause?

In the United States, the average age for menopause is 51; however, in recent times, the number of women entering menopause at 40 years old or less is increasing. This can be really challenging and frustrating if you were not ready for menopause or if you were planning to have kids because menopause signifies the end of your fertile years.

Menopause can occur prematurely due to genetics, medical procedures, or autoimmune disorders. Other conditions could cause early menopause like;

Premature ovarian failure; happens if mysteriously, the ovaries prematurely stop releasing eggs affecting the levels of estrogen and progesterone. This is called premature ovarian failure if it happens before 40. However, unlike menopause, it's not always permanent.

Induced menopause; occurs once you get your ovaries surgically removed for medical reasons such as endometriosis or uterine cancer, or surgeries like hysterectomy (removal of the uterus) or damage to the ovaries due to things like chemotherapy or radiation.

Note: You shouldn't waste all your time trying to figure out which stage you are in during this normal aging process. Instead, focus on why you're feeling unwell, having symptoms and how you can solve your menopausal issues.

The question you might be having now might be; does the onset of premature menopause have any symptoms? And is there a way to prevent it?

That's what we will discuss next.

Signs You Might Be Heading Towards Premature Menopause

Premature menopause has the same symptoms as normal menopause. When your ovaries start producing less estrogen, you may experience hot flashes, you may start missing periods, or notice irregularities in your period. You may also experience breast tenderness, fatigue and insomnia, mood swings and mild depression, vaginal dryness, loss of bladder control, and drying of the skin.

If you begin noticing two or more of these symptoms, especially irregular periods coupled with hot flashes and mood swings, you pay your physician an immediate visit so he or she can run tests to determine if you are going into early menopause and make useful recommendations for what you can do to halt the process.

Natural Ways to Prevent Premature Menopause

Nobody likes going into menopause too early especially if you are still looking forward to having kids. The strategies below can help you prevent premature menopause:

Consume a Lot of Antioxidants

Menopause is a sign of aging; therefore, if you figure out a way to slow down your body's natural aging process, you will also delay your menopause.

Toxins are very notorious at speeding up the aging process. Too much toxins in your body makes you age fast. To detoxify your body, you have to consume plenty of antioxidants.

Cranberries, raspberries, strawberries, blackberries, broccoli, red grapes, pecans, carrots, grapes, beans, olive oil, artichokes, beans, and dark chocolates are common foods that have very high antioxidant properties. Include these in your diet as much as possible.

Exercise Regularly

Regular exercise helps improve your blood circulation, prevent obesity, and keep your body healthy and young. As soon as you hit 30's, you should not skip workouts because during this time, your body requires extra help to keep you healthy and in good shape. The healthier your body, the less likely you are to go into premature menopause.

Use the Right Beauty Products

Some beauty products are not good for you because they contain harsh chemicals that speed up your aging process and upset your hormonal balance. You should start going for natural beauty care products, and avoid those that contain parabens and artificial fragrances.

You should also drink a lot of water and include lots of fruits and vegetables in your diet so you do not necessarily need too many beauty products to look radiant and beautiful.

Ease up on the Alcohol and Tobacco

Smoking and drinking excessively sets you up for premature aging and early menopause thanks to the pollution and high toxic load. It may also cause other health problems such as heart diseases and cancer. If you have a smoking or drinking addiction, look around for help maybe from healthcare professionals, addictions anonymous programs, or psychologists.

Take Phytoestrogens

Include food items high in phytoestrogens in your diet. Foods such as walnut, flaxseed, barley, rye and soybeans contain phytoestrogens that can boost your depleting estrogen levels and subsequently delay premature menopause.

It is very important to note that after menopause, you cannot conceive because at that point, your ovaries have stopped producing eggs. Therefore, if you still want children, you should keep an eye on the potential signs of premature menopause and use the tips above to delay your menopause until you get to the natural and appropriate age for menopause.

So what about the natural menopause; does it have its own signs and symptoms? Let's discuss these next.

Menopause Symptoms

How can you be sure, you are experiencing menopause? Let us look at menopause symptoms.

Hot flashes, night sweats, and insomnia

Hot flashes are probably the very first menopausal symptom you'll experience. Most women approaching menopause (perimenopausal) experience hot flashes that usually last 2-4 minutes. You usually suddenly start feeling heat from your face spreading to your upper body and then all over, with a bit of sweating and blushing, often followed by chills and shivers as your body tries to regulate temperatures. Some women have severe hot flashes while others mild with some experiencing them while still having their periods while others when their menses stop. It's not yet known why hot flashes occur but scientists feel the core of this problem is in the hypothalamus (base of the brain) and the brains thermoregulatory center as they try to react to estrogen withdrawal.

You may have hot flashes every hour of the day/night or once after a couple of days. Hot flashes are often associated with insomnia and heart palpitations. Estrogen boosts serotonin; a chemical that helps you sleep and prevents depression plus increasing GABA (brain stuff that makes you feel calm and good), while progesterone helps balance estrogen. Therefore, abnormal progesterone levels, cause insomnia and mood imbalances.

Unsurprisingly, women with intense sleep disturbances are normally moody and grouchy the following day. When hot flashes occur frequently during the day, you may feel uncomfortable and embarrassed while at night, you may have unrelenting insomnia, which could lead to irritability, fatigue, depression, anxiety, and concentration problems (may even lose focus on job-related tasks). These symptoms are more linked to chronic sleep disturbances than menopause in itself.

You may occasionally experience hot flashes during premenopausal phase- don't take this as a sign of an imminent menopause though. Some of us will have hot flashes for more than a year- if untreated, they last for a few years but some (5-10%) women will have them past 70. Obese women are more prone to hot flashes as well as women who smoke and live a sedentary lifestyle.

Irregular or skipped periods

You will experience many changes in your normal menses. As you approach menopause, production of progesterone and estrogen declines and ovulation stops. This decline in progesterone shortens your cycle length (count from the first day you get your menses to the first day of your next period). For instance, a cycle length of usually 27-30 days may reduce to 22-26 days and, as your menses become somehow irregular, with 'cycles' differing by three to five weeks apart, declining progesterone may also shorten your period-. Your menses may last for fewer days and even get lighter or heavier. Some women may start spotting before their normal menstrual flow begins. All these changes are due to the falling levels of progesterone and estrogen. As menopause progresses, you could even skip a period but, test to confirm you aren't pregnant.

Urinary inconsistency/bladder control issues

Urinary inconsistency is rather common among menopausal women which makes you find it hard to hold your urine long enough to reach the bathroom. You may suddenly get an urge to urinate or your urine could leek during exercise, coughing or sneezing. It normally starts or worsens during perimenopausal because the bladder tissues and its supporting structure depend on estrogen.

Low sex drive

Lose of sexual energy during perimenopausal and menopausal phase is a complicated phenomenon that may or may not be linked to the simple hormonal changes. Besides the loss of estrogen, there is loss of testosterone (another hormone made by ovaries) which plays a key role in sexual desire. Quite a number of things could cause you to lose your sexual energy, such as, depression, low energy levels, and family or work pressure and complicated relationship with your sexual partner. Many women who have experienced very satisfying sex well into their 40s and 50s who suddenly lose interest in sex. However, you could also feel much freer and sexier after menopause-after all you can't get pregnant but, watch out for STDs.

Vaginal dryness and atrophy

Low estrogen causes a decrease in blood flow to the vagina and vulva and reduces the amount and quality of vaginal lubrication. In the cause of time, the vagina suffers degenerative changes (atrophy) that make your vaginal wall shorter and narrower especially you've not had sex for years. Generally, atrophy develops 5-10 years after the start of menopausal hot flashes. Moreover, the vagina dries because its lining is not making enough mucus. The urethra (bladder outlet tube) also experience similar changes. This may cause urinary tract infections (UTIs) due to bacteria overgrowth.

Additional symptoms

Thinning hair, itching under skin, short-term memory loss, reduced breast size, joint and muscle aches, and headaches can also occur due to estrogen loss among other reasons like aging.

However, since we're different, not all of us experience all these symptoms. In fact, some women don't have hot flashes as their first symptom.

Long-Term Health Problems Related To Menopause

Since your estrogen levels dwindle during menopause, you may start experiencing a number of health problems.

After menopause, you may suffer from conditions such as:

Osteoporosis

Your body is always crashing old bones and replacing them with new healthy bones. Estrogen aids in regulating bone lose and when you lose estrogen during menopause, you lose more bone than is replaced. Therefore, your bones may become weak and fragile leading to a condition known as osteoporosis. Consult your doctor to see if you are at risk and seek treatment. Also, use the bone health tips I'll offer later.

Malfunctioning bladder and bowel

Pelvic floor muscles weaken due to lose of estrogen. Because these muscles control your bladder and bowel, their weakness may reduce your ability to hold or control your urge to visit the toilet. In addition, your bladder could lose elasticity causing frequent urination and significant weight gain can further weaken your pelvic muscle worsening this situation.

Increased wrinkling

Hormonal changes affect skin physiology. This is because estrogen stimulates fat deposits, which are then redistributed and stored in our abdomen, thighs and buttocks. Consequently, we lose the supportive fats in our face, neck, arms and hands causing sagging and wrinkles. Moreover, your breast may lose fat deposits causing them to sag and flatten.

Heart disease

After menopause, women are prone to heart disease due to changes in estrogen levels and aging. Age could come with possible weight gain (our body stores fat so it becomes harder for you to lose weight) and other problems like high blood pressure, which put you at risk of heart disease.

Eye problems

Hormonal changes during menopause can cause vision problems and even cataracts.

Now that you have all the basics about menopause, let's look at a number of simple effective ideas to help you cope with the troubling menopausal symptoms and lower the risks associated with these serious post-menopausal conditions.

How To Deal With Menopause Symptoms

Let us look at how to deal with menopause symptoms by learning how to take care of your adrenal glands.

Take Care Of Your Adrenal Glands During Menopause

Poor glandular function is a major contributor to your hot flushes and sleepless nights. When our ovaries stop making, progesterone, estrogen and testosterone, the adrenal glands and fat cells take over. The adrenal glands are located right above your kidneys and they produce hormones that help us deal with stress among other bodily functions. Therefore, for a very busy woman, the adrenal glands works at full capacity and to load them with the extra work of producing more hormones is the last straw. That's why many women suffer from hot flashes when going through stress.

You can eat various foods to boost the functioning of our adrenal glands. Top foods and herbs for good adrenal health include:

Take foods rich in vitamin C

Compounds in vitamin C (bioflavonoids) have been shown to reduce hot flashes and help skin elasticity by increasing collagen, which can help with bladder problems and vaginal dryness.

Foods rich in vitamin C are citrus fruits, strawberries, tomatoes, cabbage, broccoli, kiwi fruit, rock melon, and sweet red peppers.

Take foods rich in vitamin B5 and B6

These vitamins have compounds that help ease stress on adrenal glands.

Foods rich in vitamin B5 and B6 are soybeans, brewer's yeast, sunflower seeds, eggs, avocado, and fish.

You can also support your adrenal glands using amazing herbs such as:

Ginseng

Ginseng is also known as an adaptagen because it helps the body adjust to stress. Ginseng works by increasing dopamine and serotonin, which is your brain's 'feel good' chemicals boosting your moods and sleep. In addition, it is energizing; thus, it is good to take the morning after a sleepless night with a busy day ahead. The recommended ginseng dose is 800mg to 2 g a day. It's advisable that you take ginseng with food to prevent nausea that occurs when taken on empty stomach. However, avoid taking it in excess or for more than 3months.

Withania (ashwagandha)

In addition to being an adaptagen, it reduces cortisol (which causes stress). It is also relaxing as well as a powerful aphrodisiac (boosts sex). Recommended dose of 500 to 100mg twice or thrice a day (however follow instructions on the supplement). It is advisable to take the herb at night and in the morning.

Licorice root

The special acids in licorice root help nourish the adrenal glands relieving depression and nervousness.

Sage

Sage is a phytoestrogen that also helps reduce sweating and hot flushes. It is often taken as tea.

Take phytoestrogens (plant estrogens)

Phytoestrogen are nutrients that naturally occur in plants that act similar to estrogen in our bodies. Phytoestrogens work by binding to the estrogen receptors in our cells helping to balance hormones and this in turn helps in reducing hormonal symptoms. Phytoestrogens work by also slowing cell growth and preventing inflammation. If you're one of the many women out there who dread the health risks of synthetic hormones used in the usual hormone therapies, consider phytoestrogens as an alternative. Here are its main sources:

Phytoestrogen foods

Foods rich in phytoestrogen are flax seeds and other oil seeds, soybeans, fermented soya milk and flour, peas, lentils, tofu, pumpkin seeds, nuts, fennel, apples, parsley, celery, alfalfa and whole grains especially millet and rye.

Phytoestrogen herbs

Some popular herbs that are considered phytoestrogens include; Black cohosh, Red clover, and licorice root.

We should probably borrow from our Asian sisters who evidently have fewer incidences of osteoporosis, heart disease, and cancers of the colon breast and womb, due to consuming diets rich in phytoestrogen. In addition, these women apparently don't get serious hot flashes and night sweats like their western counter parts.

Therefore, when you consume a diet rich in phytoestrogen, you get various health benefits including relief from menopausal symptoms and less risk of the so-called "western diseases". Therefore, take large amounts of phytoestrogen in foods or herbal supplements (remember to consult your doctor first).

The other thing you need to care for is your liver.

Care For Your Liver

Looking after your liver is another key aspect in hormonal health, especially during menopause. There are several ways the liver is linked to hormonal health. First, it helps to process and distribute hormones into your blood stream where they perform their tasks of sending signals to your body and tissues. Secondly, it assists in eliminating excess hormones from the bloodstream and ships them to be expelled from your body. Therefore, it's quite involved in hormonal balance. However, if you overload your liver with too much detoxification tasks, it may not work at its best, which can worsen menopausal symptoms. Therefore, if you don't want to overwork your liver quit coffee, cigarettes and alcohol (stimulants), as they trigger hot flashes. Take healthy alternatives like water or green tea instead. Cut out sugar, junk food and avoid environmental chemicals (e.g. chemical cleaning products, sprays, fumes etc), since most packaged foods may contain chemicals that overburden your liver.

Then support your liver function by taking plenty of water (at least 8 glasses a day), and give it antioxidants to help in the cleansing process. Fruits and vegetables are rich in antioxidants.

In addition, many herbs support the liver, the major ones being milk thistle and globe artichoke.

Next, we will discuss the relationship between blood sugar levels and menopause.

Your Blood Sugar Levels And Menopause

Balanced blood sugar levels highly depend on what you eat or don't eat. When you eat sugary foods and simple carbohydrates, they are quickly digested and converted into glucose, which causes sharp spikes to your blood sugar levels, which is often followed by a sharp dip that can leave you feeling tired, grumpy, and craving for more starchy or sugary snacks that only worsen your situation. In addition, the excess glucose is stored as fats or converted to energy.

It is important to note that sudden rise and fall of sugar levels has been shown to cause many other problems in the body. Apart from causing weight gain, taking refined carbs and sugars can also be the root cause of your agonizing periods and menopause symptoms. Cutting down on refined sugar and carbs has been shown to reduce some menopausal symptoms like irritability and mood swings. Sugar not only causes major highs and lows in energy and mood but, it also disrupts insulin, a hormone that is closely linked to all hormones in your body including testosterone and estrogen and also helps keep the blood sugar at normal levels. Therefore, balancing your blood sugar can really help stabilize your energy and moods.

Here are some simple ideas that can help prevent blood sugar imbalances:

Eat a healthy breakfast

Start your day with veggie-protein rich breakfast. Missing your breakfast will destabilize your energy and mood levels.

Eat less but often

We need fewer calories as we age. In addition to cutting back on sugar, watch the fat in your diet. Only eat unsaturated fats found in lean meats, wild fish and vegetable oils (olive, coconut etc). Take 5-6 small portions of food per day to have energy throughout your day (three modest meals and 2 healthy snacks will do). Also, ensure that your plate has more veggies than carbs.

Include protein in each meal

Proteins have slower energy release, which ensures you don't experience blood sugar spikes. Great protein sources include foods such as meat, eggs, legumes, nuts and dairy. The solution is variety and good combination of protein and energy sources.

Eat Foods high in fiber

Fiber is found in almost all fresh vegetables and fruits especially asparagus, collard greens, eggplant, broccoli, turnips, squash, and beets. Whole grains like whole wheat, brown rice, sorghum, barley, oats and pseudo grains such as quinoa and spelt are also full of fiber. Take these foods because fiber takes time to digest and this in turn keeps your blood sugar stable. In addition, they keep you fuller for longer so won't have the cravings.

Minimize or rather cut off foods such as white rice, white bread, white pasta and all other white flour products which have practically zero fiber causing blood sugar imbalances.

The other thing you must do as you go through menopause is to protect your bones.

Protect Your Bones

Your bone density starts decreasing during menopause. Therefore, increase your intake of minerals like magnesium, Calcium, and nutrients like vitamins D and K to maintain your bone density. Let us see how these minerals and nutrients help with menopause.

Magnesium

Magnesium helps with mood swings, anxiety and irritability as well as bone strength. Foods rich in magnesium include leafy green veggies, nuts, seeds, kelp, oyster, shrimp, and avocados.

Vitamin D

It assists in absorption of calcium and vitamin K and limits osteoporosis and type-2 diabetes. Low levels of vitamin D are linked to bowel disease, poor immune function among other things. Just bask 15 minutes a day under morning or late afternoon sun to get your dose of vitamin D or, take vitamin D supplements.

Consider taking other vitamins and minerals necessary for healthy bones such as vitamin E (also good for vaginal dryness and flushes) and zinc. Opt for a supplement that has a combination of minerals and vitamins.

Avoid foods high in phosphorous

Phosphorous is found in food such as; red meat, processed food as well as fizzy drinks. Phosphorous is not good because too much phosphorus in your diet speeds up the loss of minerals such as magnesium and calcium from your bones. Reducing sodium (salt), animal protein, and caffeine can enhance calcium storage.

Choose alkaline foods

Take plenty of fruits vegetables, seeds, nuts and unsweetened yoghurt to help prevent lose of calcium from your bones.

Eat foods high in magnesium and boron

These minerals are essential for bone replacement thus helping lower your risk of osteoporosis. Good sources of boron are pears, apples, grapes, raisins and dates.

Do weight bearing exercise

You should work those muscles and keep your bone sturdy. I'll talk more about this in the exercise section.

The next aspect that you ought to be careful about to help cope with menopause is sleep.

Get Adequate Sleep

When it comes to sleep, quality matters more than quantity. What you feel when you wake up tells a lot about how you slept. Often the cure to your sleep difficulties and daytime fatigue is found in your lifestyle choices and daily routine.

Here are some ideas that you can experiment with to sleep better:

Optimize your bedroom environment

The first step is to make your bedroom an optimized ideal environment for sleeping. Here is how:

*Plug your phone charger in an outlet far away from your bed to avoid grabbing your phone while lying down. Doing this stopped me from watching YouTube or checking Facebook before I fell asleep. In fact, watching bright screens 1-2 hours before bedtime disrupts sleep.

*Wear a sleeping mask and keep the curtains drawn to make your room as dark as possible. Once your room is full optimized, set your reminder for bedtime.

Commit to a consistent bedtime and wakeup time

Try to go to sleep and wake up at the same time each day. Doing this helps reset your body's internal clock and optimizes your sleep's quality. Pick a bedtime when you're really tired to avoid tossing and turning. Prepare some minutes before your bedtime and then when the time comes, switch off the light, close your eyes, focus on your breath rhythms and let sleep take over you.

Take smart naps

A critical aspect in dealing with menopausal symptoms such as anxiety and all other sleep-related symptoms is taking a 20-

minute nap every early afternoon. Longer naps can interfere with your sleep at night. After you've had lunch, take a nap. Set 20-minute alarm on your phone, lie on your back with your eyes shut. Don't try so much to fall asleep; instead, focus on breathing in and out. Even if you don't fall asleep, you'll feel refreshed and calm every time after your alarm goes off.

Fight after-dinner drowsiness

If you feel sleepy way ahead of your set bedtime, get up and wash the dishes, call a friend or prepare clothes for the next day or anything else mildly stimulating.

Drink warm milk

Warm milk is an ancient remedy for insomnia. A glass of milk anytime of the day helps tame tension. This is because milk contains an amino acid known as tryptophan, which aids in production of serotonin which boosts your mood and promotes your well-being.

Next, I'll cover relaxation techniques that you can do before bed to help you sleep better among other things.

Effective Relaxation Techniques

Sometimes we are so caught up in our lives that we've no time for relaxation. Getting enough rest will lessen menopausal symptoms such as anxiety, stress, and insomnia among others. Take some time to calm your mind using any of the following techniques:

Deep breathing

1. Lie on your back keeping your body relaxed. Place your hands on your stomach and close your eyes.

2. Take deep slow breaths in and out and make each breath deeper than the previous.

3. Continue doing this until you fall asleep.

Doing this for just 5 minutes will significantly affect your heart rate and blood pressure.

Progressive muscle relation

Lie on your back with your eyes closed. Tense your toes as tightly as possible release after 10 seconds. Tense the rest of your muscles. Work your way up to your knees, thighs, stomach, chest, buttocks, cheeks, hands and finally roll your shoulders around. Relax after you work on each muscle.

Visual imagery

Visualize a serene restful place. Close your eyes and start imagining a calming place or activity. Focus on how relaxed this place makes you feel. Go back there whenever necessary. Visiting this place more and more will help you fall asleep easier.

Yoga

Yoga is a powerful antidote for insomnia and stress. Research has proven that if done regularly, yoga lessens menopausal symptoms. You can take a yoga class but here is a simple pose to help you wind down:

Corpse pose

Do the following:

Lie on your back. Slightly stretch out your arm and legs. Rest your palms on the floor. Think of good and positive things. Stretch out any tension in your limbs. Imagine that you're very heavy and being supported by the floor. Do this for around 5 minutes.

Medication

Another great way of dealing with your everyday stress and getting quality sleep is meditation.

Try this:

1. Find a quiet place and sit on a chair with your back straight.

2. Put one hand on your abdomen.

3. Concentrate on your lung sensations as you breathe in through your nose and out through your mouth.

4. Feel your stomach rise and fall beneath your hand. Do this for 10 minutes.

This will help clear any worries in your mind.

Massage

Massage is an old healing trick that still does wonders. With a regular massage you, feel calm and deeply relaxed even way after your massage is over. Consider having aromatherapy massage (uses essential oils).

Take a little chocolate

Taking loads of chocolate for relaxation is a universal truth. When you take chocolate, your brain muscles relax and this helps reduce anxiety and stress. Choose organic raw unsweetened chocolate and bite occasionally during the day to keep your sugar level stable.

Use lavender

This amazing anti-inflammatory herb relaxes your cells and reduces mind inflammation and this helps with, stress and anxiety.

1. Fill an infuser with lavender oil and put in your room or buy lavender fragrance and spray it in your room or keep a bottle of it nearby.

2. Wear a lotion scented with lavender or take lavender pills

The other thing you can do to ease menopause symptoms is being physically active.

Exercise

Daily vigorous physical activity has been proven to relieve stress as well as ease menopausal symptoms such as hot flushes and night sweats, improve sleep and balance hormones. In addition, regular exercise limits loss of muscle mass and weight gain, which are common side effects of menopause. The Center For Disease Control (CDC) agrees that a healthy woman should have a minimum of 150 minutes of moderate physical activity a week.

Here are some effective exercise ideas you can consider:

Cardio

An aerobic activity that utilizes your larger muscle groups and maintains your heart rate is a win. You have no limit for cardio as jogging, walking, biking, and swimming are all considered as weight bearing exercises. As a newbie, consider starting with 10 minutes of light activity then slowly increase your work out intensity to at least 20 minutes a day as it become easier.

Strength training

This workout minimizes your risk of osteoporosis and other bone problems. These exercises are vital because they'll help in building your bone and muscle strength, boosting your metabolism and burning body fat.

While at home, opt for resistance tubing and dumbbells. In the gym, either free weights or weight machines will do. Choose a level hard enough to tax your muscles in about 12 repetitions then gradually increase your intensity.

Dancing

Who said exercise can't be fun! Having a calories burning session in your routine is fun and good for you. If you do prefer running on the treadmill then consider taking a dance class. Dancing keeps you flexible and builds muscle. You can even dance to your favorite music in your bedroom.

Vigorous chores

Vigorous house/yard work that increases your heart rate and uses your larger muscle groups like, glutes, squads, and core work wonders (halfhearted dusting doesn't count). For a beginner, you can start with 10 minutes of light activity then go from there. Sweep, trim fences, mow the lawn, or do any other relevant thing you can think of.

You can also use essential oils to ease menopause symptoms.

Use Essential Oils

Essential oils (liquid plant extracts) have healing properties. They can be beneficial during menopause owing to their soothing, harmonizing and balancing effects on the mind. For instance, sage oil is the most effective essential oil for relief from menopausal symptoms like hot flashes. Furthermore, Roman chamomile oil reduces stress while peppermint oil can help in cooling your body from hot flashes.

I recommend the following oils for menopause; sage, roman chamomile, geranium, rose, lavender, peppermint and thyme

How to use

Vaporize: Add 6-9 drops of preferred essential oil to water inside the top of your vaporizer.

Body rubs: To reconnect with your femininity do this 'ritual' daily. Add 6 drops of your preferred essential oil to 12 ml jojoba oils. Apply to your body in circular motions. Start from your feet and work your way up towards your neck

Aromatic tissue: Add 1-3 drops to a tissue or cotton ball then inhale.

In bath water: Add 6 drops of preferred essential oil to a teaspoon of sweet almond before you put in your warm bath water.

Ingest: Soak sage in lemon juice and take two teaspoonfuls before bedtime to fight the night sweats. Seek advice from an expert before ingesting any essential oil.

Note; Test if you're sensitive to an essential on a soft part of your hand plus always dilute with a vegetable oil (such as sweet almond, coconut oil, olive oil etc.) to avoid skin reaction.

The next part of the book will focus largely on how to deal with specific challenges that you are likely to face during menopause. We'll start with hot flashes.

Dealing With Menopausal Hot Flashes

Hot flashes are probably the most annoying symptoms you have to deal with during menopause. That sudden feeling of heat coupled with sweats and a flushed face happens because of the blood vessels closest to the surface of your skin dilating to cool off.

You may have these hot flashes for the rest of your life or for just a few months. You can prevent hot flashes by staying away from things that may trigger it such as smoking, stress, alcohol, caffeine, wearing tight clothing, exposure to heat, and eating too spicy foods.

You can also reduce the symptoms and effects of hot flashes by taking the following steps:

Wear Cotton Nightwear

'Night sweats' are so called because they happen more at night. If you wear a lightweight nightwear to bed, it allows easier passage of air through your body and reduces the hotness and sweats.

Use a Chill Pillow

To feel cooler, you can use a pillow filled with cooling materials such as ice blocks or water.

Use an Air conditioner

You should also consider improving the temperature in your room by installing a fan or air conditioner to help you stop feeling hot.

Try Breathing Exercises

Along with exercising every day, you should also do deep breathing exercises for about 15 minutes every day or whenever you feel the hot flashes coming. Deep breathing helps calm you down and reduces the symptoms of hot flashes.

Use Natural Herbs

The following herbs have proven very helpful at reducing hot flashes:

Red Clover: The extracts from the leaves of red clover can help to reduce hot flashes.

Dong Quai: Dong Quai, commonly called Female ginseng, is a traditional Chinese herb that helps reduce hot flashes. However, women who suffer from blood clotting or fibroids should not use it since it may cause various complications.

Ginseng: Ginseng helps you sleep better and much more comfortably through the night, which ensures the hot flushes do not keep you up at night.

Evening Primrose Oil: Evening primrose oil is also a great remedy for alleviating menopausal inconveniences including hot flashes and night sweats.

The other thing you may specifically want to deal with is sex during menopause. We will discuss that next.

Menopause and Sex: Reviving Your Sex Drive After Menopause

Having a low sex drive is one of the challenges you may face after menopause; you may not feel as 'sweet' as you used to and may become less sensitive to sexual arousal.

The main cause of this is the reduction in testosterone and estrogen levels in your body, an after effect of menopause. These two hormones contribute significantly to sexual drive because the estrogen hormone is responsible for promoting the supply of blood to the vagina so that the vagina becomes more sensitive to penetration, touching, or stroking. Estrogen also promotes vaginal lubrication, another factor that is extremely important for sexual enjoyment. Without adequate lubrication, your vagina becomes too dry and penetration or touch becomes painful instead of enjoyable.

On the other hand, testosterone is responsible for increasing libido in women. Testosterone is to women what Viagra is to men: it improves your sexual drive. During menopause, your body produces less testosterone; this is the cause for your decreased sexual drive.

Solutions for Menopause-Induced Vaginal Dryness

If your vagina is too dry for, and during sex, sex becomes a painful experience instead of being an enjoyable one. You can use some of these tips to increase vaginal lubrication after menopause:

Use a Lubricant

You can use a water-soluble lubricant such as K-Y Jelly or Astroglide to improve lubrication of your vagina before sex.

Please stay away from non-water soluble lubricants especially Vaseline. These types of lubricants can easily weaken condoms and cause them to tear up during sex, thus expose you to risks like sexually transmitted diseases.

Use Vaginal Moisturizers

Some moisturizers are specially designed for lubricating the vagina. Some common brand names include Luvena or Replens. You can use this daily to improve moisture in your vaginal area.

Vaginal Estrogen Therapy

You can talk to your physician about prescribing topical creams and oral medications that can help increase the production and supply of estrogen to the vagina. Some common brand names include Estrace, Alora, Premarin, Evamist, Vagifem and Estratab.

How to Improve Your Sexual Drive after Menopause

After menopause, your sexual drive may not necessarily change. In fact, in some cases, your sexual drive may heighten. However, in many cases, because of the reduced testosterone supply, after menopause, most women experience a reduced or nonexistent sexual drive.

Here are a few ways to improve your sexual drive and keep your partner from becoming sexually frustrated:

Improve on Your Confidence

After menopause, your body may start looking different and you may not feel as sexy as you used to, which is one of the reasons why your sexual drive may decline: because you do not want your partner to notice these changes. It is important that you eat healthy foods and take good care of yourself so that you can look good and maintain a healthy self-esteem and confidence in your body.

Exercise Regularly

It is common knowledge that exercise increases your libido thanks to the increase in blood flow. Make sure you exercise regularly. You should also engage in Kegel exercises; kegels are a very effective way to strengthen the vaginal walls so you can enjoy sex.

Spend More Time on Foreplay and Oral Sex

Compared to your pre-menopausal days, after menopause, your body shall responds slowly to sex. Hence, you and your partner may have to spend more time in foreplay before penetration. Extended foreplay shall help you get in the mood and increase arousal. Oral sex is also an effective way to stimulate the clitoris, which plays a very significant role in helping you achieve orgasms.

Experiment and Spice up Your Sexual Life

Now is the time to introduce new things into your bedroom. You can try exploring erotic videos, sex toys, or any sexual fantasies you and your partner have. This makes sex less boring and naturally improves your desire for sex.

Try Natural Aphrodisiacs

Aphrodisiacs can help boost your libido and desire for sex.

You can try natural aphrodisiacs such as Cacao, Fenugreek, Spices like Cinnamon, Nutmeg and Ginger, Dates, and Shatavari. Ayurveda practices have used all these for thousands of years and each has individually proven very effective at boosting female libido.

Communicate With Your Partner

Talk to your partner about what is happening within your body and how you can change your sexual routine. Let your partner know what is painful and what is comfortable for you so that you can get your partner's full cooperation; otherwise, your partner may not even have a clue of what is going on within your body.

The key to enjoying sex during and after menopause is to be confident, avoid overthinking things, or stressing yourself. Allow your body and mind to relax and be innovative. If you do this, you may actually notice your sex life improving to a point where it's better than before you hit menopause.

The other thing we will specifically deal with is urinary incontinence.

Dealing With Menopause-Induced Urinary Incontinence

After menopause, because of significant reductions in estrogen production in your body, the lining of your urethra becomes thinner. The urethra is the short tube that transports urine from the bladder out of your body and when it thins, urine may begin to leak out. Aging may also cause your pelvic floor muscles to weaken, which may also cause involuntary urine leakage.

During menopause, you are likely to experience two major types of incontinence:

1: Urge Incontinence

This usually happens when your bladder muscles become irritated or overly active. This would then cause frequent urination, a sudden urge to urinate, and urine leakage if you cannot get to the toilet fast enough.

2: Stress Incontinence

Weakened pelvic floor muscles are the major cause of stress incontinence. If you experience urine leakage when you are sneezing, lifting objects, laughing or coughing, it is probably because of your pelvic floor muscles becoming too weak to hold in urine.

Stress incontinence can happen before you hit menopause; it may also worsen after menopause if you already have it.

Here is how to deal with these problems.

Effective Solutions for Urinary Incontinence after Menopause

Loss of control over your urine can be very embarrassing especially in cases where you mistakenly wet yourself in public. Doing the following shall help reduce urinary incontinence and improve your grip over your bladder activities after menopause:

Reduce Alcohol and Caffeine Consumption

Alcohol and caffeine are diuretics that cause your bladder to fill up faster. Hence, you should avoid them, which will lead to a significant reduction of stress on your bladder.

Train Your Bladder

You can train your bladder to only urinate at specific times of the day and hold urine more. In this strategy, you shall only urinate at preplanned times daily so that your bladder becomes stronger. You would be surprised at how smart your body can be and how quickly it can respond to training. Have you ever noticed that sometimes, the urge to urinate becomes stronger as soon as you get home or in the toilet? This is just an example of how your brain can control your bladder. You can take advantage of this and use it to control your bladder.

Lose Some Weight

If you are overweight, you should try losing some weight because excess weight puts undue pressure on your muscles and bladder. Losing weight helps reduce this pressure.

Do Pelvic Floor Exercises

Pelvic floor exercises are a very great and long-lasting solution for urinary incontinence. You can expect to start seeing results within 9-12 weeks and the results are usually permanent.

Physicians would usually recommend that you try this before recommending surgery.

Kegel exercises are the most effective types of pelvic floor exercises; they involve contracting and relaxing your pelvic floor muscles. Many people do not get results from Kegel exercises because they fail to do it correctly. Below is the correct way to practice kegels for optimum results

Locate the Right Muscles: You need to find your pelvic muscles, which you can do by stopping your urine midway. Try doing this a few times until you discover the exact location of your pelvic muscles.

Choose a Comfortable Position: The position you decide to choose is up to you; you can decide to sit or lie down, but it helps to start out with lying until you master the technique.

Expand and Contract Your Pelvic Floor Muscles: Start by tightening your pelvic floor muscles as though you want to stop your urine halfway, count from 1-10 very fast and release. After releasing, count 1-10 again and tighten again. Repeat three times and do it at least 10 times every day. Make sure you do not hold your breath during the exercise; otherwise, you shall be flexing the wrong set of muscles (buttocks or abdominal muscles).

If you try all of these without any desired results, you should talk to your physician who may prescribe medications or surgical procedures to correct urinary incontinence.

Next, we will discuss hormone replacement therapy.

Hormonal Replacement Therapy for Menopausal Women

One of the quickest ways to find relief from your menopausal stresses is through Hormonal Replacement Therapy (HRT). This therapy has governmental approval and can eliminate most menopausal problems including insomnia, hot flashes, and vaginal dryness. It can also help prevent Osteoporosis.

We have already discussed how the absence of, or reduction in the production of some hormones in your body is responsible for most of the symptoms you have to deal with during menopause. Menopausal Hormonal Replacement Therapy involves artificially introducing these hormones into your body as a way to alleviate the inconveniences you feel. During Hormonal Replacement Therapy, Estrogen and Progesterone hormones are some of the hormones injected into your body as a short-term treatment.

Hormonal Replacement Therapy usually serves to replace the vital hormones your body no longer makes because they are extremely important. Estrogen not only improves fertility, it also helps increase the assimilation of Calcium in your body and increase good blood cholesterol.

Progesterone and Estrogen usually come as a pair because without Progesterone, Estrogen may increase risks of Endometrium, a cancer of the lining of the Uterus. The cells from the endometrium are supposed to leave your body during your monthly periods but since you are no longer menstruating, the cells may build up in your endometrium and subsequently cause cancer.

What Type of Hormonal Replacement Therapy is Most Suitable for You?

There are different types of hormonal replacement therapy:

1: Progestin/Estrogen/Progesterone

In this therapy, you shall receive a synthetic form of Progesterone along with doses of Estrogen and Progestin. This is therapy is usually ideal for women whose uterus is still intact.

2: Estrogen Therapy

This type of therapy is ideal for women who have had a hysterectomy and the Uterus has removed. In this therapy, you could receive estrogen in the form of a pill, skin patch, gel, or vaginal ring.

The Benefits and the Risks of Hormonal Replacement Therapy

Although HRT seems like the easy way out, it is not suitable for everyone because in some instances, it comes with potential risks that may be severe than the menopausal inconveniences you were trying to alleviate in the first place.

The Benefits

The major benefit of this therapy is that it helps get rid of most of the menopausal symptoms you feel including poor libido, vaginal dryness, hot flushes, and night sweats. It also prevents your bones from deteriorating and reduces stress levels by preventing insomnia and sleep disturbances.

The Risks

Hormonal Replacement Therapy may have some very serious side effects. The hormones introduced into your body are synthetic hormones, not natural. Therefore, they can cause conditions such as cancer, blood clotting, bloating, nausea, vaginal bleeding, headaches, mood swings, breast swelling, or tenderness. When on hormonal replacement therapy, you may also notice an increased weight gain or digestive problems.

The benefits of hormonal replacement therapy certainly outweigh the risks but if you suffer from any of the following conditions: stroke, pregnancy, cancer, heart diseases, or liver diseases, you should avoid hormonal replacement therapy

Conclusion

We have come to the end of the book. Thank you for reading and congratulations for reading until the end.

You need to remember that menopause is a normal aging process that you can experience without having to go through hell. Consider applying what you've learnt before or during menopause in order to have a smooth transition.

Finally, if you enjoyed this book, would you be kind enough to leave a review for this book on Amazon?

That would be much appreciated.

Also, do not forget to download my bonus menopause check list!

Thank you and good luck!

Dr. Melissa Keane

Made in the USA
Lexington, KY
25 October 2017